The Simple Diet

Did you ever wonder why there are so many diets and diet books on the market? That is because everyone thinks there is a gimmick or a science to losing weight, but weight loss is actually very simple. Hence, this diet is called *The Simple Diet*.

If a person thinks about it, the three things that cause weight gain are junk food, white food, and sugar. All other foods are fine in any quantities that people choose, including fat, as long as it is the good, monounsaturated fat. The truth of the matter is that bread is actually much worse than fat, because fat only has 4 calories per gram, but bread has 9 calories per gram.

Therefore, the thing to do to lose weight is to curtail the three things I mention above. Junk food does not actually have to be abolished—just eat some once a month. Bread does not actually have to be abolished—just eat two servings of white foods a day, any out of the three, but no more. Sugar, on the other hand, should be eliminated. Switch to a sugar substitute.

People have told me how much they love bread and potatoes, but, believe me, they do not love you. It may seem like they are good because they may seem to have fiber, but the average slice of bread only has 2 grams of fiber per serving, and the same is true of potatoes.

Exercise is important, and it should be cardiovascular, not yoga, with weight-bearing, especially for women over 40. When a person lifts weights slowly instead of jerking them, then her muscles will not bulk-up like a man, and she can gain muscle mass. The thing to do is to exchange fat for muscle. A woman should put on 10 – 20 pounds of muscle to control her weight and raise her basal, or resting, metabolism. The other good thing about muscle mass is that having it stops cravings.

Water should, of course, be consumed, and it should be consumed before a person becomes thirsty. Also, instead of drinking coffee first thing in the morning, a woman should have 16 ounces of water first thing in the morning, because the body has accumulated toxins and become dehydrated overnight.

This is the essence of the diet. People will see a dramatic change when they stop eating six or more white food servings a day, and when they limit junk food to only once a month. Not having eight teaspoons or more of sugar every day will also help put a woman over the top on *The Simple Diet*.

All other foods can remain the same as before, except for animal fats, which cause heart disease and arteriosclerosis. Eat olive oil as proscribed earlier.

The average person who is obese has 4 – 8 servings of the three bad foods a day. If a person reduces from four servings to two a day, that amounts to about 400 calories saved in a day, or about 12,000 a month, for a loss of 3 pounds a month. This is good weight loss that is not in the danger area.

As it regards other foods, meat is actually not a poison, and it builds muscle on the body, not fat. Vegetables and fruits are necessary for bowel health, and 40 grams of fiber provide ideal bowel health. Milk controls blood sugar, cutting cravings. Learn what the various kinds of salads are, and eat these instead of white foods. There is Waldorf salad with apples and walnuts, garden salad, pasta salad with whole wheat pasta for one of your two servings a day, Cesar salad, Cobb salad, fruit salad, and more, all of which will be delicious when you keep rotating between them.

My doctor told me to walk 4 miles a day, but it may be different for you. Consult with your doctor. Although people think that they should park farther and walk, this is still not far enough to raise the heart rate, a necessary task for cardiovascular health. Ask your doctor how high you should raise your heartbeat during exercise. It is approximately 40 beats per minute for a 30 year old, and 20 for a senior.

Organic foods are nice, but not required. It is also not required to skip protein, and fish and eggs are necessary proteins for brain health and for obtaining the full complement of amino acids that the body needs. Eat more protein if your hair is thin or has bald spots.

Other diets use points, which are not necessary here, because the offensive items will be cut from the diet. Measuring is also not necessary, because fruits and vegetables really do not cause any harm. If desired, fruits like grapes can be limited. Specific vegetables do not have to be consumed, except for green, leafy vegetables and the red and purple antioxidant vegetables, with yellow and orange vegetables for vitamin A.

Here are also some things to do to compliment weight loss:

* Get your teeth cleaned
*Cut any perm-damaged or heat-damaged hair. Get rid of plastic brushes and chemical (inorganic) shampoo/conditioner for vitamin/herb-based products.
*Get rid of chemical make-up and use organics, like Physician's Formula™
*Take care of your feet. See a podiatrist. Eliminate spiked heels and vary heel types, especially heel width, buying new shoes as appropriate
*Take care of your skin. Use non-comedogenic moisturizers, and use cleansing and toning masks, including mud and apricot scrub. Stop using bar soap on your face unless it is natural soap

My dieting history includes The Atkin's Diet, fat-free diets, Jenny Craig, and high-protein diets. The high-protein diet was not effective, because I could only eat chicken breasts.   Jenny Craig did not enable me to cook and eat my own foods, which I love to do, and I cheated.   The fat-free diet caused me to lose weight too fast, making sagging skin and breasts that looked like bananas.   And, The Atkin's Diet was not to my liking because it called for complete elimination of junk food and soda.   By the way, you can have sodas on this diet, but not more than one a day if they are regular sodas.   Aspertame has been removed from some colas, so they are safe to drink again.

Intelligence is simple.   Thus, *The Simple Diet*.   A woman does not need all those charts, all those medical studies, or all those rules in order to lose weight and keep it off.
Try this diet!!!

Weight Promenading^{tm} is my trademark weight routine for gaining muscle mass without bulking. It is called, 'promenading', because it includes movements like dancing. Here is a description of the various dances:

Wrist promenade

Hold a two-pound weight in each hand. Twirl the weight in the right hand like a baton. Do for 20 seconds, and then switch to the left hand for 20 seconds. Rest, and then repeat 9 more times.

Torso promenade

Stand with feet shoulder width apart, and hold a ten-pound weight in each hand, with arms spread about a foot outward from your sides. Twist to the right, then to the left. Do this for about 30 seconds, rest, then repeat 19 more times.

Chest promenade

Lie on your back, with a ten-pound weight clasped in your hands and held above your chest with arms straight. Work the weight like a fulcrum, moving it up towards your face, then back down towards your crotch. Rest, and repeat 9 more times.

Arm promenade

Stand with feet shoulder width apart. Hold a ten-pound weight in each hand, with arms resting at your sides. Lift the right arm up perpendicular to your side towards the head. Then, repeat with the left arm. Rest, and then repeat 11 more times.

Neck promenade

Stand with feet shoulder width apart. Hold a five-pound weight behind your head, with arms bent at the elbow perpendicular to the head. Move the weight up, then down, parallel to your neck. Rest, and then repeat 9 more times.

Leg promenade

Stand with legs shoulder width apart.   Hold a ten-pound weight in each hand, with arms resting at your sides.   Lunge forward with the right leg, bending it at the knee, then step backwards to a standing position. Repeat with the left leg.   Alternate with each leg 9 times more.

Appendix: Starter Recipes

Some of these recipes call for organics for those who like them, but regular ingredients can also be used. They will help you get your mind off the three, deadly foods, and onto good eating!

1.   Simple Rich Granola Bars (simple to make, and simply rich!)

Note: Check product labels before purchasing ingredients to make sure that you have exactly the ingredients called for below! (To save money, shop around, and buy in bulk!)

2 cups of unprocessed honey
1 cup of natural peanut butter (stirred first, to mix in the peanut oil)
4 cups of plain, rolled oats
1 ½ cups coarsely chopped plain walnuts, i.e., without preservatives
1 tbl extra-virgin olive oil

In large saucepan, over low heat, bring honey to a boil. Stir in peanut butter until melted. Turn off heat, but leave pan on the burner. Stir in oats, one cup at a time. Mix-in walnuts. Turn into a 9"x 13" pan greased beforehand with the olive oil. Cover with plastic and chill about 1 ½ to 2 hours. Cut like brownies with a butter knife to avoid scratching the pan. Makes approx. 24 bars.

2. Organic Popcorn (see below for amount needed [about 2/3 cup for a large, 2 quart pan])

3/4 cup unprocessed honey
½ cup Natural Peanut Butter (mix first with its natural oil)
1 cup chopped plain Walnuts

Coat a large pan with olive oil.   Cover the bottom of the pan with organic popcorn kernels (put in just enough to cover the bottom of the pan with a single layer of kernels).   Place over high heat with a lid until kernels begin to pop.   Decrease to 3/4 heat.   Pop by shaking back and forth over heat until kernels stop popping.   Immediately remove from heat and place popcorn in a large mixing bowl.

Wipe out pan with a paper towel.   Add honey and heat to a boil over low heat.   Add peanut butter and dissolve.   Remove from heat.   Let cool 5 minutes, then add walnuts.   Cool for another 5 - 8 minutes to prevent melting of popcorn.   Mix thoroughly by parts into popcorn. Chill in refrigerator for about 45 minutes.   Makes 8 - 10 servings.

3.   Quick Organic Black Soybean Soup

2 tbl extra virgin olive oil
1 can plain, cooked organic black soybeans
½ fresh lemon
4 large organic fire-roasted peppers
1/3 coarsely-chopped onion
6 medium cooked, peeled tomatoes (in the can is O.K. if they contain nothing but tomatoes in their own juice)

        Chop onion and fire-roasted peppers.   Saute in 2 tbl extra virgin olive oil until onions are clear.   Place soybeans, tomatoes, and sauté mixture in a 3 qt saucepan.   Slice and add lemon juice.   Heat, stirring occasionally, for 10 minutes.   Serves 2 – 3.

4.   Quick, Thick Black Bean Soup

2 12 oz cans plain, cooked black beans (preferably Gia Russa or Goya brand)
12 oz refried beans (Taco Bell brand has no fat, sugar, artificial color or preservatives!)
8 strips of bacon (Well done, but not dark or crispy) and the fat from them
1 tsp chicken bullion
1 ½ cups crushed tomatoes

Fry bacon on medium heat until brown on both sides.   Place black beans, including sauce, in a 4 qt saucepan.   Stir in chicken bullion and heat on medium low to dissolve.   Stir in refried beans a tbl full at a time.   Add crushed tomatoes and mix in.   Heat entire mixture for 10 minutes.   Serve with 2 bacon strips crisscrossed over the bowl.   Serves 4 – 6.

5.   White Chocolate Cookies

2 eggs, preferably Eggland's Best
1 cup butter
4 squares white chocolate
8 tbl Splenda
2 cups whole-wheat flour, or amount needed to achieve correct consistency
1 tsp baking soda

Preheat oven to 325.   In a small saucepan, melt butter over very low heat.   Add white chocolate to butter when butter is partially melted.   Let both just become melted, without bubbling or boiling.   Once chocolate and butter are completely melted, transfer to a medium-size bowl.   Add splenda.   Stir until splenda dissolves.   Add eggs and blend.

In a separate bowl, combine flour and baking soda.   Gradually add flour-soda mixture to butter mixture, stirring completely after each addition.   When finished, mixture should be the same consistency as peanut butter cookie dough.

Drop by rounded tablespoonfuls at least 1" apart on an ungreased cookie sheet.   Bake for 8 to 10 minutes.   Makes 18 cookies.

Variation #1: Add ¾ cup uncooked oatmeal, and decrease flour accordingly (by approx. 1/2 cup).   Increase sugar to 12 tbl Splenda.

6.   A Pasta Salad

1 pkg tri-color spelt pasta
½ large green bell pepper
6oz large pitted black olives
12 baby carrots
1 8oz pkg organic provolone cheese

Dressing:

1 Large Pinch Red Raspberry Leaves
1 Large Pinch Flaxseeds
3/8 Cup Extra Virgin Olive Oil
1/8 Cup Red Wine Vinegar

    Cook pasta until al dente.   Drain and place in a bowl.   Toss with 2 tbl Olive Oil to prevent sticking and let cool for about 10 minutes.   Cut carrots into 4ths and add.   Core and wash pepper, cut into strips and dice, add to bowl.   Drain Olives, cut into halves, and add.   Dice and add cheese.   Measure and mix ingredients together to make dressing in a separate cup. Add to salad and toss.   Chill for 15 minutes to cool and let flavors mix.   Makes 8 - 10 servings.

7.   Quick Avocado Crabmeat Salad Spread

1 can pink or white organic crabmeat
1 very ripe organic Avacado
1 tbl canola oil mayonnaise

Drain crabmeat, remove paper cover, and place in a medium-sized bowl. Wash, peel, and mash cut Avocado--cut it around the seed into slices, then dice and mash. Mix with crabmeat. Add mayonnaise and mix. Spread onto the bread of your choice, and add bean sprouts, making a sandwich. Makes 2 - 4 sandwiches.

8. Steamed Balsamic Chicken for One [All ingredients assumed to be taken as Organic to prevent redundancy in listing of ingredients.]

1 sliced free-ranging chicken thigh
12 - 16 whole fresh green beans
1/4 large yellow bell pepper
½ tsp ginger
2 small cloves garlic
2 tbl balsamic vinegar

Fill a 2-quart saucepan half full with water. Turn on high heat. Wash and slice chicken, trimming off the excess fat. Clean and pick beans without snapping. Clean and slice pepper in long strips. Place these three ingredients in a medium-large hand strainer and hook over pot when water has come to a boil, with the chicken at the bottom and the pepper strips on top. Cover with a lid a little larger than the pot. Chop the garlic and add. When chicken is about half done (when tested with a fork), pour vinegar over the chicken, turn, and cover again. Dish is done when chicken is done. Serves one.

9.   Black-Eyed Susan's

10 hard-boiled eggs
1 tbl dry mustard
5 tbl mayonnaise
1 tsp celery seed
1 tsp garlic salt
black cumin (topping)

Boil eggs in an extra-large pot with enough water to cover eggs until an egg, when lifted out of the pot with a serving spoon, dries immediately. Pour-off most of the hot water and flood with cold water. Let sit for 5 minutes, then crack and peel. Halve eggs, removing yolk into a small bowl. Mash egg yolks with a spoon until pea-sized. Add mustard and mix. Add mayonnaise and cream mixture with spoon. Stir-in celery seed and garlic salt, mixing thoroughly. Put egg mixture in rounds (i.e., not flat-topped but heaping) back inside whites. Sprinkle each half with about 10 black cumin seeds (a tiny pinch). Chill for an hour, then serve. Makes 20 black-eyed Susan's.

10.   Cucumber Bacon Salad for One

1 medium cucumber
½ yellow bell pepper
3 dtrips dlab bacon

Dressing:

   2 large cloves garlic
   1/8 tsp flax seeds
   1/8 tsp red raspberry leaves
   1 tbl extra virgin olive oil
   1 tsp balsamic vinegar
   1 tbl bacon drippings

   Wash cucumber with a tiny dot of soap so that you can eat the skin as well.   Cut in half lengthwise and then cut each half into 1/6" slices and place in a bowl.

   Fry bacon, turning often so that it will cook evenly and be medium golden brown all over.   While bacon is frying, chop garlic into crosswise slices (i.e., along the clove's shorter dimension, or vertical slices.)   When bacon is done, remove to paper towels to soak up extra grease, and sautee garlic in the rendered fat.

   Remove garlic into a cup or bowl for making the dressing.   Add warm bacon drippings, olive oil, and vinegar.   Stir.   Add flax seeds and red raspberry leaves, mixing thoroughly.

   Combine cooked bacon, broken into 1" long pieces with cucumber and ½ bell pepper, cut in half again crosswise and then into slices.   Mix-in dressing.   Makes one salad.

11.   Loin Chop Pasta Sauce for Two

2 center-cut 1-inch thick pork loin chops
1 28-oz can whole, peeled tomatoes
3 tbl julienne sun-dried tomatoes in olive oil
4 cloves fresh garlic
canola oil for frying

Place sun-dried tomatoes in a bowl and cover with water.

Fill skillet with ½ an inch of oil.   Turn on high to warm.   Wash chops.   Pat dry, and place in hot oil.   Turn flame down to medium.   Cook for 5 minutes on each side, and then remove to platter.

Drain all but a tiny bit of the oil, just enough to coat the pan.   Peel and dice garlic, and then sautee.   Place whole tomatoes in a 1-quart saucepan.   Add garlic.   Drain sun-dried tomatoes and chop.   Add to sauce,   Break up tomatoes with a spoon.   Simmer for 15 minutes. Remove bone from chops and cut meat into small cubes.   Add to sauce and cook for 8 minutes more.   Make the pasta you desire and use sauce.

12.   White Pizza

1 Boboli pizza shell, large
4 sliced onions, large
8 mushrooms
2 bell peppers, any color
12 oz mozzarella cheese
6 oz grated fontina
6 oz sliced blue cheese
1 lb proscutto

Peel and slice onions in 1/6" thick slices crosswise.   Wash and slice mushrooms, and wash, core, and slice bell peppers into strips lengthwise.   Slice blue cheese into thin slices on the small side of the block.   Place fontina and mozzarella all over shell.   Arrange vegetables and blue cheese slices on top of cheese.   Bake at 425 degrees for 15 min.   Remove and cool. Serves 8.

13.   Cornbread

¼ cup melted butter
1 cup buttermilk
2 eggs
1 cup flour
1 cup cornmeal
1 ½ tsp baking powder
½ tsp baking soda

        Combine and mix dry ingredients well.   Make a well in the center and add melted butter, eggs, and buttermilk.   Mix until just combined.   Bake at 400 degrees for 20 min, or until tester comes clean.   Cool and slice.   Serves 8 – 12.9

14.   Whole-Wheat Natural Anise Sugar and Iced Cookies

[This combination recipe is meant for making a variety of Christmas Cookies, both regular and traditional iced cookies.]

2 - 2 ½ cups regular whole-wheat flour
1 cup whole-wheat pastry flour
1 ½ tsp baking powder
1 cup organic butter [2 sticks]
2 eggs [Eggland's Best or other Organic (i.e., from free-ranging hens) Eggs]
1 ½ cups Splenda (36 packets)
1 tsp pure vanilla

Natural Anise Flavor:
        3/4 cup Fresh Licorice Root
        3 cups water

Natural Anise Icing:
        natural Anise Flavor (as above, prepared as described below)
        ½ cup organic butter, softened
        2 - 2 ½ cups powdered sugar

        Place water and Licorice Root in a 2-quart saucepan.   Place on high heat.   When water comes to a boil, reduce heat to low, and let simmer until liquid is brown and about twice as thick (i.e., half its original volume).   Remove from heat and strain in a very fine (the grade of a tea strainer) metal strainer.   Place over flame again in a smaller pot and simmer to 2 - 3 oz (1/3 - 1/4 cup) of liquid.   Remove from heat and set aside.

        Preheat oven to 350.   Measure flour into a large bowl, sifting with a slotted spoon as you measure.   Make a well in the center, add baking soda and stir together.   Melt butter in a small saucepan on the lowest heat/setting until half-melted.   Remove from heat.   Melt completely by stirring with a wooden spoon.   Place in a separate bowl.   Add sugar and vanilla, then eggs, mixing well after each addition.   Gradually add flour mixture (i.e., in small parts, mixing well after each).   If (some of) remaining ½ cup of flour is needed, add and mix.

        Turn dough onto a floured surface, rolling to 1/6" thickness.   Use cookie cutters, maximizing the dough area for the shapes used.   Leave plain, without colored sugar or decorations, for icing. Place on a lightly greased cookie sheet (with olive oil) and bake for 12 - 15 minutes, or until firm and golden brown.   Repeat these steps until dough is exhausted.   Ice. Makes 2½ - 4 dozen cookies, depending upon the (size of) the cutters used.

Icing:

Soften and cream butter.   Add pre-made anise syrup.   Add powdered sugar in small parts and blend, until exhausted.

Icing:

Cream softened butter in a small bowl, after preparing anise flavor.   Gradually add powdered sugar, and cream into butter.   Add flavor and mix well.   If cookies are cool, refrigeration of the icing is not needed.   Ices 12 - 18 cookies.

15.   Flamingo Shrimp

½ yellow bell pepper [Organic preferred]
½ tsp whole Flax Seeds
½ tsp Hyssop
½ tsp Blackberry Leaves
3/8 cup Expeller-Pressed Extra-Virgin Olive Oil
8 - 10 large shrimp

    Wash, core, dry, and divide pepper.   In a large, deep skillet, heat olive oil on very low.
Cut pepper into wide strips (about ½"), then dice.   Sautee in pan for 2 minutes.   Place whole,
washed, and deveined shrimp in with pepper after 2 - 3 min (after peppers start to glaze) and
increase heat to medium low.   Add flax seeds, hyssop, and blackberry leaves.   Stir. Cook,
turning shrimp when bright orange, until both sides are done.   Makes one serving.

16.   Lemon Grass Tempura

30 Medium Shrimp, Shelled and Deveined (fresh or frozen--thaw.)
1 Large (Organic) Orange Bell Pepper
[The next three ingredients are approximate:]
2 tbl Lemon Grass
2 tbl Flaxseeds
3 ½ Cups (Organic) Whole Wheat Flour
1 Small Saucepan
2 Cups [Organic Expeller Pressed] Olive Oil

        Prepare and rinse shrimp.   Place olive oil in the saucepan and heat over medium high flame. While oil is heating, make flour mixture in parts, in order to cook shrimp and pepper in parts, with ½ tsp of lemon grass and ½ tsp of flaxseeds to ½ cup of flour.   Wash, core, and cut pepper into 1/6" strips.   Lightly roll about six shrimp and a few pepper strips in flour mixture and cook for about three minutes, or until surface of shrimp are light golden brown with an orange color underneath.   Remove and place on paper towels to drain.   Keep refreshing flour mixure and cooking ingredients in this manner until all the shrimp and pepper strips are done. Makes 4 - 6 servings.

17.   Tart Crust (Own Filling)

1 ½ - 2 Cups Whole-Wheat Flour
2/3 Cup Organic Butter
1 tsp baking powder
1/4 Cup Water

      Measure flour into a medium-sized bowl.   Stir-in baking powder and mix thoroughly with a mixing spoon.   Cut-in butter until mixture resembles coarse crumbs.   Add water by teaspoonfuls, moving dough to the opposite side of the bowl with a fork each time, until it's moist and formed into a ball.   Divide equally in two, and roll out onto a floured surface (the same whole-wheat flour) until dough is slightly bigger than the pie pan.   Pick-up dough, folding in half (you should be able to do this if dough was not made too moist and the surface was properly floured) and place into bottom of pan by placing the fold in the middle and gently releasing each half without stretching.   Add desired filling and place other crust on top.   Bake as usual.

18.   Oatmeal Raisin Bars

2 eggs
2 sticks butter
2 cups flour
2 cups oatmeal
1 cup raisins
1 tsp baking soda
¾ cup sugar
¾ cup packed brown sugar

Preheat oven to 350.

Melt butter on low in a small saucepan without browning.   Remove from heat, and transfer to a mixing bowl.   Gradually add sugar, mixing as you go.   Do the same with the brown sugar.   Add eggs and mix.

In a separate bowl, combine flour and baking soda.

Gradually stir in flour mixture.   Measure and gradually add oats.   Fold in raisins.

Place mix in a 9" x 13" pan, spreading evenly with a spatula.

Bake at 350 for 25 minutes, or until golden brown on top and set in the middle.   Cut into 1" squares.   Makes 25 bars.

19.   Turkey Chowder

1 bay leaf
½ tsp oregano
½ tsp garlic powder
½ tsp onion powder
½ tsp basil
1 red bell pepper
1 large can of kernel corn (12 – 16 oz.)
2 turkey legs
turkey back meat
2 turkey wings
2 turkey thighs
   3 tbl olive oil

Fill a 4 quart saucepan 2/3 full with water.   Add turkey.   Bring to a boil.   Turn down to simmer, and skim pot.   Add spices.   In a separate frying pan add olive oil and heat on medium. Chop and core pepper, and sautee.   Add to pot.   Remove bones from meat with a spoon when tender.   Add corn.   Cook for 15 minutes more.   Makes 10 –12 servings.

20.   Chicken with potatoes

1 roasting chicken
4 large white or red potatoes
1 tbl paprika
1 tbl sage
1 tbl garlic salt
2 cups water

Preheat oven to 325.   Wash chicken and remove any stray feathers.   Remove giblets.
Place in a medium roasting pan, breast side up.   Add 2 cups water.   Sprinkle spices over
chicken.   Place in oven and bake for ½ hour.

While chicken is baking, wash potatoes thoroughly and cut into quarters, leaving skin on.
After ½ hour, add potatoes around chicken.   Bake for another hour.   Serves 6.

21.   Broiled steak with broccoli

2 New York Strip Steaks, 12 oz. each
½ tsp black pepper
½ tsp garlic powder
½ tsp oregano
12 broccoli florets

    Preheat broiler to 425.   Rinse steaks and pat dry.   Divide spices between steaks, sprinkling over them.   Place in broiler.

    Meanwhile, add 2 cups water to a 1 quart saucepan.   Wash broccoli and place in water. Bring to a boil.   Turn down flame to medium and cover.   Cook for 5 minutes more, then remove from heat.

    Steaks should be done.   Place on plates with broccoli.   Serves 2.

22.   Chicken with Mexican Rice

4 chicken thighs
2 cups white rice
1 large red bell pepper
½ tsp garlic
1 large can kernel corn (12 – 16 oz.)
4 cups water

Wash thighs and check for feathers.   Sort rice, and place in electric skillet on high with water.   Add thighs skin side down.   Cook for 7 minutes, then add diced pepper and corn. Cook until rice is done.   Serves 4.

23.   Coffee Cookies

2 tbl instant coffee
1 stick butter
¾ cup sugar
1 ½ cup flour
1 tsp baking soda
1 egg

Preheat oven to 350.   In a mixing bowl cream softened butter.   Gradually add sugar and mix,   Add egg, then coffee.   In a separate bowl, combine flour and baking soda.   Gradually fold into mix.   Place by tablespoons on a greased cookie sheet and bake for 10 – 12 minutes.   Cool on rack.   Makes 2 ½ dozen cookies.

24.   Egg Salad Sandwich

2 diced boiled eggs
2 slices whole wheat bread
¼ tsp dry mustard
3 tbl ,mayonnaise
¼ tsp garlic salt
2 leaves lettuce
1 slice avocado

In a small bowl, mix diced eggs, mustard, spices, and mayonnaise.   Place lettuce on one slice of bread.   Place egg salad over lettuce and spread out.   Top with avocado, and other slice of bread.

25. Fruit Shake

½ cup strawberries
½ cup raspberries
8 oz milk
2 tbl honey

Place berries in a blender and blend until pureed.   Add honey and milk, and blend until mixed.   Serve in a tall glass for one.

26. Home Fries

4 large potatoes

1 medium onion
1 large bell pepper
½ tsp garlic salt
½ tsp oregano
½ cup canola oil

Wash potatoes thoroughly and cut into fries.   Heat canola oil in a large skillet.   Dice bell pepper and chop onion.   Place potatoes in pan and cook, turning when golden brown.   After turning once, add onion and pepper to pan, with spices.   Brown on the other side, and remove from heat.   Serves 4.

27. Sausage Meatballs

2 lb sausage links
1 large bell pepper
1 large onion
½ tsp sage
½ tsp oregano
½ tsp basil

Remove sausage from casings and place in a bowl.   Dice pepper and onion.   Add to sausage along with spices and combine.   Roll sausage into 1" balls.   Fry in a large skillet until browned, turning to ensure that all sides are done.   Makes 16 meatballs.

28. Lemon Bars

2 sticks butter, softened
4 large lemons
3/4 cup sugar
1/2 tsp baking soda
2 1/2 cups flour
2 medium eggs

Preheat oven to 350. Cream butter in a large mixing bowl. Gradually add sugar. Add eggs and beat. Using a grater, take zest of lemons and mix in. Juice lemons and add to mix. In a separate bowl, combine flour and baking soda, sifting together. Gradually fold in flour to the butter mixture. Turn into a 13" x 9" pan, spreading evenly out to sides of pan. Bake for 20 - 25 minutes until a tester comes out clean. Makes 20 bars.

29. Old-Fashioned Apple Sauce

30 granny smith apples
1 tbl cinnamon

Wash apples, but do not peal.   Core and cut into quarters.   Place in a large (8 quart) pot., and cover with water.   Bring to a boil. then simmer.   Add cinnamon.   Cook until apples turn into sauce, about 1 1/2 - 2 hours.   Serve warm.   Makes 12 - 15 servings.

30. Pork Chops (to be served with old-fashioned apple sauce)

4 bone-in pork chops, large
1 tsp garlic salt
1 tsp oregano
1/2 tsp black pepper
1 tsp sage
8 tbl flour
3/4 cup cooking oil

Heat oil in a large skillet until hot. Wash chops. Coat chops with a mixture of the flour and spices placed in a bowl. Fry chops until golden brown on each side. Remove to a plate covered with paper towels. Serve with apple sauce.

31. Chili Con Carne

3 lb stir fry beef
1 pkg (12 - 16 oz) dry kidney beans
1 22 oz can tomato puree
1 22 oz can whole tomatoes
1/2 tsp garlic salt
1/2 tsp oregano
1 bay leaf
pinch of ginger
1/4 tsp red pepper
2 tbl cooking oil

Wash and sort beans.   Place in 6 quart pot, just covering with water.   Boil for 2 minutes, then let set for an hour.
In a separate, 2 quart saucepan, combine puree and spices.   Add crushed tomatoes with juice, and break up with a spoon.   Simmer for 20 minutes, then set aside.   Cook beef in oil until brown (about 10 minutes), then set aside.

Add a quart of water to bean pot, and cook beans until tender.   Combine with sauce and beef, and simmer for 30 minutes.   Makes 8 - 12 servings.

32. Egg Nog

8 egg yolks
1 pint Burbon
1 pint heavy cream
4 cups half-and-half
1 tbl nutmeg

Place half-and-half in large punch bowl.   Beat in egg yolks.   Add Burbon.   Beat cream until stiff and spoon on top of mixture.   Sprinkle with nutmeg.   Makes 8 - 12 servings.

33. Waffles

2   cups flaxseed fllour
1 1/2 cups buttermilk
1 tbl baking soda
1 large egg

    Preheat waffle iron to medium high.   In a medium bowl, combine flour and baking soda. Add buttermilk and stir. Add egg. Pour mix onto griddle of iron. Bake as usual. Makes 4 - 6 waffles.

34. Tuna with Homemade Relish

1 12-oz can tuna
4 slices whole wheat or multigrain bread
4 leaves lettuce
1/2 medium onion
4 sweet baby pickles
3 tbl mayonnaise

Chop pickles and place in small bowl. Chop onion and add. Drain tuna and add. Stir in mayonnaise and mix thoroughly. Place bread on plates with lettuce leaves on one face and spread tuna mixture on top. Cover each with other slice of bread and cut in half diagonally. Makes 2 servings.

35. Beef Gravy

6 tbl flour
1 bay leaf
1/2 tsp oregano
1/2 tsp basil
1/4 tsp black pepper
2 16 oz cans beef stock or equivalent stock from roast

Heat flour in a large skillet over medium heat, stirring with a wooden spoon continuously until medium brown.   Add stock, and turn heat to low.   Add spices, and stir.   Let simmer for 15 minutes or until gravy tickens.   Serves 4 - 6.
For chicken gravy, use 1/2 tsp sage, 1/2 tsp garlic salt, and 1/2 tsp paprika instead, with 32 oz chicken stock.

36. Grilled Cheese Sandwiches

1/2 stick butter
 4 slices whole wheat or multigrain bread
8 slices cheddar or monteray jack cheese
4 slices medium tomato

    Place 4 slices of cheese between each two slices of bread, with 2 slices of tomato inside each on top of the cheese.   Place butter in large skillet on medium low heat.   Place sanwiches in pan, and let brown on both sides, 5 minutes each side.   Makes 2 sandwiches.

37. Turkey Stuffing

1 large bag cubed stuffing bread
1/2 tsp garlic powder
1/2 tsp sage
1/2 tsp oregano
2 1/2 cups turkey stock
1 medium onion
2 branches of celery stalk
1 medium green bell pepper

Preheat oven to 325.   Wash and chop vegetables.   Place bread cubes in a large casserole.   Add stock and mix.   Combine spices and vegetables.   Bake at 325 until top is crusty.   Makes 6 - 8 servings.

38. BBQ Ribs

2 bottles of your favorite barbecue sauce
2 tbl black pepper
2 tbl garlic powder
2 tbl onion powder
2 racks pork ribs

Preheat oven to 175.   Wash ribs, and place in large roasting pan.   Divided spcies between two racks and rub into ribs.   Place in oven for 2 hours.

Remove to barbecue grill.   Place flame on medium and brush on barbecue sauce,   Grill until sauce is set.   Serves 8- 10.

39. Venison Roast

1 tsp white pepper
1 tsp ground cumin
1 tsp onion salt
1 tsp dried parsley
1 3 lb venison tenderloin roast

Preheat oven to 225.   Make sure all of the fat is trimmed from venison.   Wash and sprinkle with spices.   Place in a baking dish and roast until tender.   Serves 6 - 8.

40. Eggs and Onions

3 eggs
1 large onion
1/4 tsp garlic salt
2 tbl canola oil

Cut onion in half and slice onion into medium thick slices.   Place canola oil in a large skillet on medium.   When oil is hot, add eggs and scramble.   Add onions and spice and let cook together until onions are translucent.   Serves 2.

41. Hamburger Pizza

1/2 pkg dry yeast
2/3 cup warm water
2 1/2 cups flour
2 bell peppers, different colors
1 1/2 lb ground beef, lean
1 12 oz can pitted black olives
1 large onion
1/2 tsp oregano
1/2 tsp garlic powder
1/2 tsp basil
1 22 oz can tomato puree
1 32 oz pkg shredded mozeralla cheese

Preheat oven to 375.   In a medium bowl, measure flour.   Heat water until clearly warm, and measure 2/3 cup.   Place yeast in cup and mix.   Make a well in the center of the flour and add yeast.   Add rest of warm water by small parts to bowl and toss flour to one side of bowl each time.   Form into a ball, and cover with a dishtowel.   Set in a warm place to rise for 1 hour.

In a large skillet, brown ground beef with spices.   Drain any grease and remove to seperate bowl.

In a medium saucepan, heat tomato puree with same amount of spices used for hamburger.   Let simmer to thicken.

Wash vegetables, core peppers, and slice them into rings.   Press dough into pizza pan, spreading evenly across pan.   Cover with sauce.   Distribute vegetables around pizza.   Top with hamburger, then cheese.   Place in oven for 20 - 25 minutes until cheese is melted and crust is golden brown.   Serves 8 - 10.

42. Peach Cobbler

12 large peaches
2 1/2 cups flour
1 stick butter
approx. 3/4 cup water
1/2 tsp cinnamon
1/2 tsp nutmeg
3/4 cup sugar

Preheat oven to 350.   In a medium bowl, combine flour and butter, cutting butter into flour until it resembles pea-sized crumbs.   Add water by bits, scraping dough to one side of bowl with a fork.   Form into a ball and roll to fit a 13" x 9" glass (pyrex) pan on a large sheet of waxed paper.   Place dough in pan, making sure that sides are covered.

Wash and peel peaches, cutting into vertical slices of 8 per peach.   Place in bowl and combine with sugar and spices.   Pour on top of dough.   Place in oven for 20 - 25 minutes, until peaches are done.   Serves 8 - 12/

43. Baked Apples

4 yellow delicious apples
1/2 cup raisins
1/4 cup sugar
1 ssp cinnamon

Preheat oven to 350.   Wash and core apples.   Place in a glass baking pan.   Fill cavities with raisins and sugar.   Sprinkle cinnamon over apples.   Bake at 350 for 10 minutes. Serves 4.

44. Cinnamon Toast

2 tbl brown sugar
2 tsp cinnamon
2 slices white bread
8 pats butter

Preheat oven to 325.   Place bread on a baking sheet.   Distribute 4 pats of butter each over the slices.   Sprinkle one tbl sugar over each, and 1 tsp cinnamon over each.   Bake for 5 minutes.   Serves 2.

45. Candied Yams

3/4   cup sugar
2 tsp cinnamon
2 cups water
2 large yams

    Wash and peel yams.   Cut into quarters and boil until tender.   In a separate, 1 qt saucepan combine water and sugar, stirring until dissolved.   Bring to a boil and cook down until thick.   Stir in cinnamon and remove from heat.   Place yams in sugar pot and coat. Serves 2 - 4.

46. Relish Plate

8 celery sticks
1 small jar or can pitted black olives
1 small jar sweet pickles
1/2 pkg Philadelphia Cream Cheese
2 tbl peanut butter

Wash enough celery, removing leaves, and cut stalks in half to make 8 sticks.   With the tip of a knife, fill half with cream cheese, and half with peanut butter.   Pack olives with cream cheese with same knife.   Slice pickes in half lenghtwise.   Arrange on a serving tray with olives in the middle, surrounded by a ring of pickle slices, and celery on the outside.   Serves 4 - 8.

47. Spam Treats

1 can Spam
16 Sociables Crackers
8 black olives
16 slices Monterrey Jack Cheese
2 tbl canola oil

Slice spam block in half, then into 8 slices.   Fry until golden brown in a large skillet with oil.   Just before done, melt cheese on top of each slice.   Arrange crackers on platter.   Place a slice of spam on each cracker.   top with an olvie half in the center.   Makes 4 - 8 servings.

48. Tropical Punch

16 oz Grapefruit Juice
16 oz Orange Juice
16 oz Pineapple Juice
4 oz Lime Juice
2 trays ice cubes

In a large punch bowl, combine juices and stir. Chill for 1 hour. Remove, add ice cubes, and serve. Makes approx. 8, 6oz servings.

49. Pineapple Upside Down Cake

1 can (16 - 22 oz) pineapple
3 eggs
1/4 cup olive oil
3 1/2 cups flour
1 tsp baking soda
3/4 cup sugar
1/4 cup brown sugar

Preheat oven to 350. In a large bowl, combine flour and baking soda. Make a well in the center, and add eggs. Add oil in the same well. Then, add pineapple juice and sugar, and mix thoroughly with 100 strokes. Grease a 13" x 9" pan and line bottom with pineapple slices, cutting in half if necessary. Fill spaces between pineapple with brown sugar. Pour mix into pan. Bake for 25 minutes or until tester comes out clean. Makes 12 servings.

50. Chick Pea Salad

1 can (16 oz) chick peas
1 large cucumber
2 large tomatoes
8 oz crumbled Feta Cheese
1 medium onion
1/2 tsp garlic powder
1/2 tsp oregano
1/2 tsp basil
1/4 cup olive oil
4 tsp red wine vinegar

Wash vegetables and slice cucumber and core and dice tomato. Place in a large bowl with chick peas. add garlic salt. Toss, then sprinkle with cheese. Mix dressing in a bottle with oil, vinegar, and spices. Pour over salad and serve. Serves 4.

51. Biscuits

1 stick butter
1 cup cold water
2 cups flour
1 tsp baking powder

Preheat oven to 350.   In a small bowl, measure flour.   Cut in butter until mixture resembles small peas.   Gradually add enough water, moving dough to the side with a fork each time, until a ball is formed.   Roll 1/2" thick onto a floured surface.   Place on a greased baking sheet and bake 10 - 12 minutes.   Serves 4 - 8.

52. Waldorf Salad

2 large apples
1/2 head lettuce
1/2 cup raisins
1/2 cup walnut halves
5 tbl mayonnaise

Wash, core, and dice apples. Place in a medium sized bowl. Shred lettucc and add. Add raisins and walnut halves. Add mayonnaise on top and toss until coated. Serves 2 - 3.

53. Grilled Sole

2 large sole fillets
1/2 medium lemon
2 tbl olive oil
1//2 tsp tumeric
1/2 tsp garlic powder

Preheat broiler to 425.   Wash fish and pat dry.   Coat a shallow pan with oil.   Place fish in pan.   Slice two slices of lemon for garnish.   Squeeze juice over fish.   Place slices on fish, and sprinkle with spices.   Cook for 5 minutes.   Serves 2.

54. Bean Salad

1 can (16 - 22 oz) chick peas
1 can (12 - 16 oz) black beans
1 can (16 oz) kidney beans
1 tsp garlic powder
4 tbl olive oil
1 tbl vinegar
1 medium onion

Drain beans and place in a large bowl.   Mix oil, vinegar, and garlic in a bottle.   Dice onion and add to bowl.   Pour dressing over beans.   Serves 6.

55. Pork Kabobs

4 center cut, boneless pork chops, cubed
1 yellow bell pepper
1 medium onion
1 large white potato
1/2 tsp black pepper
1/2 tsp sage
4 skewers

    Sprinkle cubes with spices.   Peel potato and cut vegetables into cubes.   Alternate potato cubes, pepper cubes, and onion cubes with pork on skewers.   Cook on medium on grill for 10 minutes.   Serves 4.

56. Apple dumplings

6 large granny smith apples
1 stick butter
2 cups flour
1/2 cup cold water
1 tsp cinnamon
1/2 small lemon

Preheat oven to 350.   Wash, core, and cube apples.   Sprinkle with lemon juice and set aside in a bowl.   In a separate bowl, add flour and cut in butter until mixture resembles small peas.   Add water by bits, moving dough to one side with fork.   Form into a ball, then roll onto wax paper until 1/4" thick.   Cut into quarters.   Transfer to a greased baking sheet. Place apples in the center of each piece of dough, sprinkle with cinnamon, and pinch around to make a dumpling.   Bake for 15 - 20 minutes or until golden brown.   Serves 4.

57. Iced Tea

6 herbal tea bags, your choice
2 large lemons
2 quarts cold water
1 cup sugar

In a large pot, bring water to a boil.   Turn off heat and add tea bags.   Let steep until water is cool.   Pour into a half-gallon pitcher.   Add juice of one lemon, and slices from the other.   Add sugar and stir.   Chill for 2 hours.   Place in glasses with ice.   makes 8 servings.

58. French Toast

1 egg, beaten
1/2 tsp vanilla
2 slices whole wheat or multigrain bread
1/4 stick butter

Place beaten egg in shallow bowl. Mix with vanilla. Run bread through egg mixture and coat. Cook in a medium skillet with butter on medium heat. Makes 1 serving.

59. Tartar Sauce

4 tbl mayonnaise
6 tsp sweet relish
1/4 tsp dry mustard

Mix ingredients together in a small bowl.   Serves 2 - 4

60. Lemonade

8 large lemons
1 cup sugar

Wash lemons.   Slice and place in a 2-quart pitcher.   Add sugar and let sit for 1 hour. Add cold water and stir.   Chill for 2 hours and place in glasses with ice cubes.   Makes 6 servings.

61. Soft Shell Tacos

1 lb. ground beef
1/2 tsp cayenne pepper
1/2 tsp garlic powder
1/2 tsp oregano
1/2 tsp basil
1/2 large bell pepper
1 small onion
1/2 head lettuce
1 large tomato
1 16 oz. pkg shredded Monterey Jack cheese
1 pkg soft flour tortillas
1 12 oz bottle taco sauce

Dice onion and pepper. Place in small skillet with ground beef. Add spices. Break up ground beef with a wooden spoon while cooking and turn until browned. Drain grease and place in a bowl. Set aside.

Shred lettuce, and dice tomato. Place in separate bowls. Place 4 tortillas on plates. Fill with beef, lettuce, tomato, and cheese, dividing evenly between the four. Add taco sauce. Serves 4.

62. Cocoa

1/2 cup powdered cocoa
2/3 cup sugar
3 cups milk
1/2 tsp vanilla

In a medium saucepan, combine cocoa and sugar.   Mix well.   Add milk by tiny parts, mixing into a paste.   Then, add remaining milk.   Stir in vanilla.   Heat on medium until hot. Serve in mugs and add marshmallows as desired.   Makes 3 servings.

63. 3 Egg Omelet

3 large eggs
1/4 diced red bell pepper
4 oz shredded cheddar cheese
1/4 tsp oregano
1/4 tsp basil
4 oz diced ham (precooked)

Beat eggs with diced pepper and spices in a medium bowl.   Heat a large. non-stick skillet until hot, then add egg mixture.   Wait until egg is almost set, then add ham and cheese on top.   Fold over in half and cook for 3 more minutes.   Serves 1 - 2.

64. Cinnamon Toast

2 slices white bread
8 pats butter
2 tsp cinnamon
4 tsp sugar

Preheat oven to 350.   Place bread on a baking tray.   Evenly distribute 4 pats of butter on each slice.   Sprinkle 2 tsp sugar on each, and one tsp cinnamon on each.   Bake for - 10 minutes or until edges of bread are brown.   Makes 1 - 2 servings.

65. Mashed Potatoes

8 medium potatoes
1/2 stick butter
1/4 tsp black pepper
1/2 tsp garlic powder
1/2 cup milk

Peel potatoes and boil in a large pot until just done by fork test. Drain, and place in a large bowl. Add butter and beat on medium with electric mixer. Add milk and mix. Fold in spices. Serve warm. Serves 4.

66. Poached Eggs

2 large eggs
1/8 tsp black pepper
1/8 tsp salt

Fill a medium saucepan half full with water and bring to a boil. Crack one egg at a time in the water and maintain state of boiling until egg is set. Remove with a large spoon to a plate and divide salt and pepper between the two egs. Makes 2 servings.

67. Cucumber Sandwiches

4 slices white bread
1 medium cucumber
1/4 stick butter, softened

    Place bread on a tray.   Remove crust.   Spread with butter.   Slice cucumber lengthwise and place 3 slices between each of two slices of bread.   Slice sandwiches on the diagonal. Serves 2 - 4.

68. Stuffed Tomatoes

2 large red tomatoes, firm
1 regular can tuna
2 tbl mayonnaise
2 tsp sweet relish
1/4 small onoin

In a small bowl, combine drained tuna, mayonnaise, relish, and diced onion, Mix well. Cut 4 verticall slits evenly spaced in top half of each tomato. Spread tomato open and stuff with tuna. Serves 2.

69. Simple Roast Turkey

2 tbl paprika
2 tbl sage
1/2 stick butter
1 large onion
1 10 lb turkey

Preheat oven to 325.   Wash turkey and check for feathers.   Remove giblets.   Rub with butter and coat with spices.   Place onion in cavity.   Cook 29 minutes per pound, or check with a meat thermometer to 170 degrees.   Cool and slice.   Serves 8 - 12.

70. Beef Roast

1 10 lb roast
2 cups water
1 tsp black pepper
1 tsp tumeric
1 tsp oregano
8 large white potatoes
6 carrots, halved

Preheat oven to 325. Wash beef and place in a large roasting pan. Add water and sprinkle with spices. Place in over and cook for 45 minutes. Wash, peel, and qusrter potatoes. Place around roast. Wash and cut carrots and place in pan. Cook until meat thermometer registers 165. Cool and slice, with potatoes and carrots on the side of the plate. Serves 8.

www.ingramcontent.com/pod-product-compliance
Lightning Source LLC
Chambersburg PA
CBHW051948280526
45789CB00009B/3220